Atkins Diet Essentials

Turbocharge Your Weight Loss with this New and Improved Version of Atkins' Classic Diet Plan

Atkins Diet Essentials
Turbocharge Your Weight Loss with this New and Improved
Version of Atkins' Classic Diet Plan

By Hanna Davis

Copyright © 2015 Softpress Publishing

Disclaimer:
This product is not intended to diagnose, treat, cure, or prevent any disease. The advice and strategies contained herein may not be suitable for every situation. This work is sold with the understanding that the publisher is not engaged in rendering medical or other professional advice or services. The publisher does not specifically endorse any company or product mentioned or cited in this document. Websites listed were accurate at the time of publishing but may have changed or disappeared between when it was written and when it is read.

No responsibility or liability is assumed by the publisher for any injury, damage or financial loss sustained to persons of property from the use of this information, personal or otherwise, either directly or indirectly. While every effort has been made to ensure reliability and accuracy of the information within, all liability, negligence or otherwise, from any use, misuse or abuse of the operation of any methods, strategies, instructions or ideas contained in the material herein, is sole responsibility of the reader.

All information is generalized, presented for informational purposes only and presented "as is" without warranty or guarantee of any kind.

All trademarks and brands referred to in this book are for illustrative purposes only, are the property of their respective owners and not affiliated with this publication in any way.

i

Table of Contents

Introduction

I want to thank you for purchasing the book, "Atkins Diet Essentials: Turbocharge Your Weight Loss with this New and Improved Version of Atkins' Classic Diet Plan".

Created by Dr. Robert C. Atkins over 40 years ago, his namesake diet plan still continues to be one of the most popular ways to lose weight to this day. And with good reason. Despite its critics, Dr. Atkins plan for controlling carbohydrate intake is very effective at helping people of all shapes and sizes lose and maintain the weight they desire.

This book is a tribute to Dr. Atkins and all the millions who have successfully used his plan to regain a healthier body and lifestyle. In the following chapters you will find a succinct outline of the Atkins Diet plan as well as many favorite recipes of those who have used this plan and lost weight to improve their health. I have done extensive research to compile this book for you and cut through all the mumbo jumbo and hype around this diet plan to bring you exactly what you need to get going today and keep you motivated tomorrow.

One last thing, as a way of saying Thank You for buying my book I have put together a **FREE GIFT** just for you!

"Atkins Diet Desserts"

This gift is the perfect complement to this book so just head over to this web address to get access:

https://tinyurl.com/3vcba4xb

Chapter 1 - Who was Dr. Atkins?

Dr. Robert C. Atkins developed a revolutionary diet plan that would help millions of people finally lose the weight they had been struggling with for years. Dr. Atkins was a cardiologist who pioneered the idea of treating medical conditions via more natural solutions rather than over-the-counter drugs and expensive, often dangerous surgeries. He stressed the importance of a healthy diet and a healthy weight as the best preventers of heart disease and diabetes. Decades ago, Dr. Atkins predicted our country was headed to a dangerous level of obesity if we didn't start curbing our eating habits. Eating habits didn't change and we are in a serious state of health concerns with our rising obesity levels. Dr. Atkins was right!

He wrote numerous books about controlling carbohydrate intake as a very effective way of controlling one's weight. His ideas made him a leader in the natural health field. People were tired of the dangerous pills that were being doled out to those struggling to lose weight. The side effects of those weight loss pills far outweighed the benefits of losing a few pounds. Dr. Atkins created a much safer approach to weight loss that has become one of the most popular diets of all time.

The diet isn't anything new. It has been around for 40 years and is still going strong. It isn't a fad or one of those diets that helps you lose 20 pounds really fast in a way that will ultimately hurt your body. Dr. Atkins won numerous awards and accolades during his lifetime for his innovative approach to staying healthy and fighting off diseases. Of course, there were plenty of people who disagreed with his methods and have continued to question his ideas more than a decade after his death.

No matter how many times people question the science behind minimizing carbohydrate intake, there are plenty of studies (more than 80) that prove it is a healthy way to eat and maintain a healthy weight. His original book, that outlined the Atkins Diet plan, remains one of the best-selling books of all time. The estate is still thriving as people hoping to get healthy without popping pills turn to the Atkins Diet for help.

Chapter 2 - Why Atkins Works

With 40 years of success, people often wonder why does the Atkins Diet work? Why does the Atkins Diet succeed where so many others have failed miserably? There have been a lot of fads and trends over the years, but Atkins is the only one that has managed to withstand the test of time, results and science. It works because nobody has been able to prove it doesn't! Quite the contrary, actually. Skeptics who are hoping to find the smoking gun that will blow this diet out of the water have failed.

Atkins is based on the idea your body will burn more fat when it is fed less refined carbohydrates. Carbohydrates are transformed into sugar during the digestive process. The excess fat generated by a diet high in carbs gets stored all over your body in that dreaded term we hate—fat.

You already know refined sugar is the ticket to obesity and numerous health problems. By limiting the amount of refined carbohydrates you eat, your body will work on burning fat, rather than wasting time and energy trying to burn through the carbs you have eaten. More fat burned means more weight lost, which is why it works!

The Atkins diet is more of a way of life. Once you have gone on the Atkins diet and reached your goal weight, you will be able to maintain your weight by loosely following the diet. It is a healthy way of eating and you will feel good when your body is in prime condition. You will know which foods you should and shouldn't eat. It is all about retraining your mind to crave the foods that will keep your body healthy.

Another reason people like the Atkins diet is the fact they are not starving while they are on the diet. You can still eat the foods you like, as long as they are high in protein and low in refined carbohydrates. Protein tends to make you feel full, which means you are going to be eating less without even really noticing. You are not regulated to soups and salads. In fact, you can eat a wide variety of delicious foods that will satisfy the carb cravings.

Because this method of eating has been around for several decades, it has been fine tuned to accommodate some of the downsides. The New Atkins Diet, which we will focus on in this book, looks a lot like the original version Dr. Atkins first introduced, but there have been some adjustments to help make the diet more effective while eliminating some of the side effects people have reported experiencing over the years.

One of the major complaints about the diet plan was the elimination of caffeine and alcohol. While it is still personal preference and there are a lot of health benefits to eliminating both items from the diet, the New Atkins allows you to have both items—in moderation. Caffeine can dehydrate you so it is important to watch your water intake. Alcohol is filled with empty carbs or refined carbs and will definitely count against the total net carbs you can consume in a day and still lose weight.

Pros and Cons of Atkins and Who Should Try It

Despite the overall safeness of the diet and the proven effectiveness, the Atkins diet is not for everybody. As with all things in life, there are some really great things about the diet and some things that are not so great. Take the time to read through this information. You should always check with your doctor before starting any diets as well.

Pros
- Ability to dine on steak, eggs, chicken and other lean meats;
- Weight loss is rather quick in the beginning;
- Flexibility in carb intake based on each individual;
- No hunger pains;
- Fairly easy to follow the diet without a lot of effort;

Cons
- Potential to increase cholesterol levels by eating the wrong cuts of meat and eating whole dairy products;
- Potential to develop kidney stones by excess urination that results in too much calcium being lost;
- Ketosis—this is normal, but it can be extreme for some people;

Who Should and Shouldn't Try Atkins

Okay, should you even bother reading this book any further? There is a possibility, although slim, the Atkins diet is not meant for you. You can certainly tweak the diet and still follow a low-carb regimen and take advantage of the health benefits. There isn't really any particular group of people who need to avoid the entire concept of the diet. Work with your doctor to tweak it to suit you and your health.

Vegetarians and Vegans will need to tweak their diet to include more plant proteins. It is also recommended vegetarians and vegans jump right into the second or even third phase of the diet. You will learn more about that further in the book.

Women who are nursing should definitely discuss the diet with their doctor. Nursing mothers need a lot of calories and carbohydrates to keep their energy up and their milk supply adequate.

You know your body. If you have tried low-carb diets in the past and discovered they didn't work or you didn't like how you felt, this may not be your ticket to weight loss. Not every diet will work for every person. There is no magic one-size-fits all weight loss cure. It is trial and error and then more trial and error as you readjust your way of eating and allow your body to catch up with the new diet. Hopping from diet to diet every month is likely to result in no significant weight loss. You have to be willing to stick it out and let your body adjust to your new way of eating. Give the new Atkins diet a chance to work. If you can, aim for a period of at least 3 months of following the Atkins way of eating. You will learn more about the diet plan and be pleased to see it isn't really a strict diet at all. You will be able to eat foods you love with the garnishments and condiments you have come to appreciate.

Chapter 3 - First 2 Weeks on Atkins

This is it! The first two weeks on the Atkins diet are exciting! What's even better is the fact you will see immediate results. You may lose a single pound or five pounds during the first 14 days. Everybody is different, but you **will** see results. That first pound or two coming off will give you incentive to stick with it and soon, the pounds will start falling away. It is exciting to weigh yourself after a few days of reducing carbs to discover you are actually losing weight.

For some, the first two weeks is the most difficult. It is essentially the crash course in Atkins and in order to really kick start the weight loss that will happen, you need to do a bit of a carb cleanse. You are going to be reprogramming your body to burn fat instead of carbohydrates. This is the key to the diet and is the ticket to dropping pounds.

It is important this part of the diet only lasts for a short amount of time; it is not the diet in its entirety. Some people go a week without carbs and decide it isn't for them and they simply cannot do it. They give up before they fully understand how the diet works. The first two weeks, which is referred to as the induction phase, are by far the toughest. You may experience some withdrawal symptoms as you flush the carbs out of your system and force your body to change the way it has been doing things.

Some of the withdrawal symptoms are as follows:
- Headache
- Nausea
- Tiredness
- Sore/achy muscles
- Crankiness
- Foggy or muddled head feeling
- Trouble concentrating

These symptoms are temporary and are just a sign your body is going through some changes. You can offset the symptoms by taking a vitamin supplement. B vitamins will help restore your energy and combat the headaches. The foggy feeling or lightheadedness can also be treated with a little extra sodium in the diet. Some chicken broth at lunch or a stir fry dish with soy sauce can help take care of that disjointed feeling. The extra sodium can also take care of any muscle aches that you may experience.

Just remember, this is only temporary!

What to Eat and What to Skip

The goal is to eat no more than 20 net grams of carbs a day. Net grams are not total grams of carbohydrates. Fruits and vegetables that contain carbohydrates, but also contain fiber are often referred to as good carbs. Good carbs don't count against your total carb count for the day. For example, if you were to eat a food that has 20 grams of carbohydrates and 10 grams of fiber, your net carb count would be 10 grams.

Fiber is insoluble by your digestive system and will be moved right through. It doesn't affect your blood sugar levels, which means the carbohydrates attached to that particular food are not going to be absorbed by the body and transformed into fat nor will they spike your blood sugar level. This gives you a little more flexibility with the foods you can eat.

Cutting your carbohydrate intake to less than 20 net grams is probably going to be a real shock to your system. Check a few labels on the things you normally eat today and you will see that is the amount of carbs in a single serving of most breads and pastas. The induction phase is designed to help your body get rid of the excess carbohydrates that your body has been holding on to and making you fat. They have to go!

These are foods you need to avoid during the first two weeks on the Atkins Diet:

- Fruit—temporary due to the sugar content
- Pastas
- Bread
- Flour
- Sugar
- Legumes (beans)
- Starchy vegetables i.e. corn, potatoes

This may seem like a huge part of your normal diet and it probably is, but you are doing this diet to change the way you look and feel. To do that, you need to change what you eat. The induction phase isn't permanent and you will be able to start eating fruits and starchy vegetables again—in moderation. During this phase, there are plenty of foods you can eat. You won't even really notice what you are cutting out when you load up on foods that are high in protein.

Foods to eat
- Red meats (avoid those that are cured with sugar, i.e. bacon and ham)
- Fish
- Chicken, turkey, duck, pheasant
- Eggs—cooked any way
- Cheese—1 serving a day which equals about 1 slice
- Low-carb veggies i.e. celery, radishes, lettuce, cucumbers
- Cooking oils—canola is best
- Butter in moderation
- Salad dressings and toppings like bacon bits, cheese, eggs, mushrooms and sour cream

As you can see from that list, the diet does not look like a diet at all. Imagine eating a lean steak with a nice salad with dressing on the side. You can eat the foods you love and still lose weight!

Personal Carb Balance

Our bodies are all a little different. One of the major benefits to the new Atkins diet program is the flexibility to find your personal carb balance. Your lifestyle will influence the number of carbohydrates you need to function and stay healthy. There will be some trial and error as you try and find the perfect number of daily carbs that leaves you feeling energetic, but also allows you to lose weight.

This part of the diet will not go into effect until the second phase of the Atkins diet program. You will know when you have found what the maximum number of carbohydrates you can consume is when your weight loss slows to less than a pound a week.

Some people may discover they can eat 60 grams of carbs a day and still lose weight while others will have to stick around 30 to 40 grams a day. The following are some of the key factors that will influence your personal carb balance:
- Age
- Gender
- Activity level
- Hormonal problems
- History of weight loss and weight gain
- Medications you are currently on

Ladies, as you are probably already aware, men tend to lose weight faster and have a higher personal carb limit. That is just a fact of life. Young people are also prone to lose weight faster while eating higher levels of carbohydrates on a daily basis. If your job involves sitting at a computer most of the day, your allowable carb number is going to be lower. If you are on your feet most of the day, like a nurse or teacher, you will be able to consume more carbs. Figuring out your personal carb balance can take a couple of months. Don't give up!

Dining Out

Do you have to sacrifice your weekly lunch date with your friends while you are on the Atkins diet? No! You can still enjoy meals in restaurants and stick to your diet. You are going to have to be a little choosier about the meals you order and you will likely need to ask the server to leave off the side of bread, rice or baked potato. Opt for steamed vegetables or a salad instead. If the restaurant serves bread before the meal, don't eat any. If you are with a group of friends who don't mind not eating bread, ask the server to skip bringing the bread basket to your table altogether. There is no need to tempt yourself!

Try these tips to help you enjoy a meal at your favorite restaurant without feeling like you need to sit and watch everybody else eat while you "starve:"

*Before leaving the house, eat a small snack. Choose something that is in line with the Atkins diet. Some sliced turkey or a small salad will help curb your appetite, but still leave you feeling like you could eat a meal.

*If it is a restaurant you are familiar with, decide what you are going to order before you get there. If you are not familiar with the restaurant, try looking up the menu online and find a meal that will not blow your diet. Most chain restaurants provide all the nutritional information, including carb counts, on each meal. This helps you eliminate the temptation to "cheat just this once" when you are looking at the menu and seeing all those delicious carb-filled dishes.

*Order that big chef salad complete with sour cream, meat, bacon bits and dressing, but skip the croutons and tortilla strips.

*If possible, avoid Italian restaurants that are heavy on pasta and pizza crusts that are loaded with carbs.

*If going out to breakfast, order omelets and other high protein dishes with bacon, sausage and eggs. Skip the French toast, waffles and pancakes.

*You have seen it a hundred times probably, but ordering a Big Mac without the bun or a quarter pounder hamburger without the bun is always your best option when eating fast food. Grab a fork and enjoy a filling meal without the carbs.

Chapter 4 - The 4 phases of Atkins

The Atkins diet is divided up into 4 phases. It is one of the only diets that helps you drop weight quickly, while teaching you a whole new way to eat. Following the outlined steps will help you drop weight and keep it off. It isn't like a fad diet that helps you drop 20 pounds in a month and the minute you go off the diet, you gain the weight back and then some. The 4 phases are crucial to losing weight in a manner that is safe and will help you keep it off for good. Although you will lose weight fairly quickly in the beginning, it is a safe diet plan. You are not starving yourself or doing anything risky that would damage your heart. It is about reprogramming your body to burn fat—like it was intended.

Phase 1 - Induction

Induction is the phase we covered in the last chapter. It deserves its own chapter because it is so crucial to the process of losing weight on Atkins. The very minimum you should do this phase is two weeks. However, if you are tolerating it well and feel great, you should try and go a whole month in the induction phase. You will drop a lot of weight rather quickly. This is an encouraging start and will give you the motivation to keep going.

During the first two weeks on the Atkins diet, your body is going to start going through something known as "ketosis." People will tell you all about this "horrible" condition, but it isn't quite as bad as it sounds.

Ketosis is the name for the condition of the body using fat instead of carbohydrates for energy. When a person is in a state of ketosis their appetite decreases. They tend to feel full as the body burns stored fat. That stored fat is exactly what you want to burn off. It is why people start to lose weight very quickly when they start Atkins. The process is fairly quick.

Now, ketosis can become dangerous if it becomes extreme. However, it is rare it would ever get to that point by following the Atkins diet. You can buy Ketone testing sticks that will tell you if the amount of ketones your body is releasing through the urine is at a dangerous level. The sticks are easy to read and will help you monitor the amount of ketones you are expelling. The ketosis will also cause your breath to smell fruity or sweet. This is the body's way of getting rid of those ketones as well. Drinking lots of water can help reduce the fruity breath. Ketosis is normal when you are eliminating the excess refined carbohydrates in the body.

Despite what many diet gurus say about eating all day to lose weight, the Atkins approach sticks with the 3 square meals a day approach with 2 healthy snacks in between. Another key is to drink lots of water and skip the soda and beer that tend to have hidden carbohydrates and sugar during the induction phase. You can reintroduce them later, but the induction phase is meant to be a total cleanse.

Phase 2 - Ongoing Weight Loss

After the first two weeks of doing the Atkins diet, or longer if you feel you can stick with phase 1 for a month, you will move into phase two. It is often referred to as the OWL phase, which means ongoing weight loss. You will still lose weight during this phase, but not as fast as you did in phase 1.

In this phase, you will add a few more carbs to your diet. Veggies and fruit return and you can even add some beans. This is the process where you will start to identify your personal carb balance. During phase 1, your daily carb goal was around 20 grams a day. You can slowly start to increase it by adding things like yogurt, strawberries, nuts and cottage cheese. It is a good idea to add the carbs back into your diet in slow increments. This will help you identify your personal carb balance quicker. You can also add in a glass of wine or a beer or two on the weekends during phase 2.

Adding an additional 5g to 10g a week is a good way to start. If you stop losing weight, it is time to back it down a bit. This phase can last for several months as you work towards your goal weight. Ideally, you will want to move on to the next phase once you are within a few pounds of your goal weight. You have probably heard and maybe even experienced dramatic weight loss that only ends up being gained right back. This happens when the diet ends and old habits are reignited.

You want to train yourself to continue to eat right without feeling as if you are on a strict diet. Good eating habits and a regular exercise plan will help you achieve your goal of maintaining a healthy weight. During the weeks you stuck with phase 1, you identified foods that were high in carbohydrates. Throughout phase 2, you will discover your personal carb balance and how much you can eat without gaining weight. Because it has probably been several weeks or even several months of counting carbs, you have become a bit of a pro at it. You no longer have to write down every bit of food you eat or look up the carb contents. You know it and have essentially learned what you can and can't eat without reading labels and putting a lot of energy into it. It is now a way of life for you.

Phase 3 - Pre-maintenance

Welcome back whole grains! Yes! You can eat carbohydrates again—in moderation! You should be right around your weight goal here. You will lose a few more pounds, but it won't be nearly as quick as it was in phase 1 or 2. You are getting into a regular rhythm now and are not really on a diet any longer. You are eating what is good for you and will help you maintain a healthy weight. You may shed a few more pounds or plateau.

This is the phase where you will be adding in a few more healthy carbs, but still avoiding white bread and pastas. You do not want to bring refined carbohydrates back into your daily diet. There is a chance that once you start reintroducing foods that are a little higher in carbohydrates than you have become accustomed to, it will spark cravings. Resist the temptation to have "just one bite" of your favorite bread. You could end up setting off a craving that will be extremely difficult to combat.

Do not sabotage all of your success. Sometimes, it is best to leave it alone. If you have managed to live months without a bite of a buttery biscuit or your favorite dinner rolls, you can do without them for good. Don't fall for the trap that one bite won't hurt. It won't hurt in the moment, but your brain is going to be demanding you give it more and more.

You will likely hit your weight plateau during this phase. If you are at your goal weight, that is fine. If you still want to lose a few more pounds, cut back on the carbs by about 5g and see if that helps. It is a fine line between giving your body too much that it will burn the carbohydrates instead of the fat and giving your body just enough.

Phase 4 - Lifetime Maintenance

Congratulations are in order if you have made it to the fourth and final phase! You hit your goal weight and now it is all about making smart food choices and keeping the weight off. Throughout the phases of the diet, you learned which foods were making you fat. Some people can eat more carbs than others. This is why it is so important to find the right amount of carbohydrates for you and your lifestyle.

You have essentially trained yourself so if your lifestyle changes, you will know when those pounds start creeping up what you need to change to take it back off. You don't have to go through phase 1 again. You can just ease up on the carbohydrates a bit. It will be much easier to choose the right foods once you have been following the Atkins way for a while. It will be second nature for you to reach for whole grain breads and pastas rather than the kind loaded with refined carbohydrates.

Chapter 5 - What to Do When You Plateau

One of the biggest reasons people give up on a diet and exercise plan is because they plateau. You are going along, losing a pound or two a week and feeling good about yourself. You are within a few pounds of your goal weight and then bam! Nothing! You cannot seem to lose a single pound even though you are sticking to the diet. It is frustrating and when you stop losing weight, you become discouraged.

Despite how irritating and depressing those plateaus are, when you hit one, it is not the time to give up. As we mentioned earlier, plateaus are going to happen when your body balances out and you are feeding it the perfect amount of food to maintain your weight. Really, those plateaus are kind of a good thing. You have just discovered how you are going to keep from gaining any weight!

If you still want to lose a few pounds and you are stuck on a plateau for a few weeks, it is time to cut out a few more grams of your daily carbs. Sometimes it is as little as 5 grams and others may have to cut 10 grams. Give yourself about a week of being on the lower carb regimen and see if the weight starts to come off again. **Whatever you do, don't give up!**

Exercise is a Must!

Along with cutting back on carbohydrates and calories in general, you absolutely must implement an exercise regimen. You cannot expect to lose weight while sitting on the couch thinking about it. Cutting carbs is great, but you want your body to burn those fat stores. The only way to do that is to get moving! You will lose weight a lot faster if you exercise regularly while reducing the amount of refined sugars and carbohydrates you eat.

When you do hit a plateau, you can cut your carbs by 5g and up your exercise by 5 to 10 minutes. Cardio is an excellent way to get your heart rate up, which is what you want to do to burn fat. If you normally walk for 15 minutes after dinner every night, make it 25 or 30 minutes.

You probably started out slow on your exercise regimen because you were overweight and didn't really have the energy or physical strength to do much more. Now that you have been steadily losing weight and eating a diet designed to keep you energized, you will likely feel better and be able to handle a more strenuous exercise regimen. It is amazing how much lighter you feel after dropping 5 to 10 pounds. You will breathe easier and feel better walking, biking or even hiking.

Don't be afraid to try some resistance training as well. You have probably heard "Muscle weighs more than fat," and you cringe at the thought of building up your muscles and packing on the pounds. Unfortunately, that phrase is not accurate. A pound of fat weighs as much as a pound of muscle. A pound of fat weighs as much as a pound of rocks. Pounds are pounds. However, the phrase is meant to explain that muscle takes up less space than fat. So, a body that has defined muscles and weighs the same as a body that is higher in fat will look leaner than the body with a higher fat ratio.

When you think about it, you could still weigh 160 pounds, but look like you weigh 140 pounds or whatever your goal is. It isn't always about the scale. You really need to calculate your Body Mass Index. This will help you figure out your best weight. There are plenty of free BMI calculators you can use to track your progress. According to the CDC, your BMI target should be between 18.5 and 25.0.

Chapter 6 - Recipes

What can you eat on the Atkins diet? You will be amazed at the wide variety of meals you can eat and still manage to lose weight. These are recipes you are probably already familiar with, but they have been tweaked a bit to reduce the carb content. Despite the adjustment, they are still delicious, filling and will leave you satisfied. The Atkins group has a large number of products on the market that are quick and easy to grab and are in line with the program. You can find flour substitutes that you can use to make some of your favorite recipes as well. Low-carb eating has become very trendy and there are plenty of companies who are creating ready-to-eat foods and various ingredients that are low in refined carbohydrates.

You can help stay on track by making some of these meals ahead of time and popping them in the freezer. When you get home after a long day of work, you won't be tempted to reach for something that is quick and already made and loaded with carbohydrates.

Breakfast

Waffles
1 cup Atkins Cuisine All-Purpose Baking Mix
1 packet granular sugar substitute
2 teaspoon baking powder
¼ teaspoon salt
1 cup half and half
1 large egg

Mix dry ingredients in a bowl. In another bowl, mix half and half and egg. Pour liquid into middle of dry ingredients and mix well. Fill waffle iron as directed by manufacturer. Recipe makes 5 waffles.

Fried Eggs and Veggies
1 tbs Coconut oil

1/2 cup Spinach
1/2 Frozen Vegetable Mix
salt and pepper to taste
3 to 4 eggs

Heat coconut oil in a skillet. Add veggies and let heat for 3 to 4 minutes. Mix in eggs and cook until done. Add salt and pepper to taste.

Sweet Potato Skillet Meal
1 lb breakfast sausage
2 medium sweet potatoes, diced
5 eggs
1 avocado, diced
handful cilantro
hot sauce
shredded cheese, optional
salt and pepper

Brown the sausage over medium heat in a cast iron or oven safe skillet. Remove the sausage (leaving grease) and add in sweet potatoes. Cook thoroughly before adding the sausage back to the pan. Crack eggs into the pan. Place the skillet into a preheated 400 degree oven. Let cook for 5 minutes. Turn the oven on broil for about a minute. Remove skillet and top with avocado, cilantro, cheese and season to taste.

Broccoli and Cheese Omelets
4 cups broccoli florets
4 whole large eggs
1 cup egg whites
1/4 cup reduced fat shredded cheddar
1/4 cup grated cheese--Romano
1 tsp olive oil
salt and fresh pepper

Steam the broccoli until it is soft. Crumble the broccoli and add in olive oil, salt and pepper. Mix well. Use cooking spray to grease a muffin tin. Spoon broccoli mixture into 9 tins. In a bowl, mix eggs and cheeses together. Pour mixture over broccoli until tins are about ¾ full. Cook at 350 for 20 minutes.

Pineapple Smoothie
1/2 Cup unsweetened almond milk
1/2 Cup Greek yogurt
2 1/2 Ounces fresh pineapple, chopped into cubes
20 whole almonds, blanched

Put all ingredients in a blender and blend until smooth

Blueberry Parfait
1/2 Cup Greek yogurt
1 granular sugar substitute (sucralose)
12 almonds
1/4 Cup blueberries

Place yogurt in a bowl and sweeten with sugar. Top with blueberries and almonds

Coconut Protein Shake
3 1/2 Ounce-weights coconut milk
1/2 Ounce-weight sugar-free protein powder (1 Tablespoon)
1/8 Teaspoon vanilla extract
1/2 banana

Place ingredients in a blender and mix well.

Lunch

Cauliflower and Bacon Chowder
8 slices center-cut bacon, chopped (half used for garnish)
1/2 small onion, chopped OR 1 teaspoon onion powder
1 celery stalk, chopped
2 garlic cloves, minced
salt & pepper
4 cups shredded or grated cauliflower (1/2 large head)
2 Tablespoons water

2 Tablespoons flour
2 cups chicken broth, divided
2 cups 2% milk
3-4 dashes hot sauce
2-1/2 cups (12oz) shredded sharp cheddar cheese, divided (half used for garnish)
2 green onions, chopped (optional)

In a small bowl, whisk ¼ cup chicken broth and the flour. Set aside. Cook bacon in a large saucepan. Remove bacon and place on a paper towel, leaving 1 tbsp of bacon grease in the pan. Add onion, celery and garlic and sauté for 5 minutes. Add cauliflower to the pan and mix well. Add in water and cover. Let cauliflower steam for 5 minutes. Pour in remaining chicken broth and turn up to high heat. Bring mixture to a boil. Slowly whisk flour and broth mixture. Turn down to a simmer, stirring frequently until chowder has thickened. Remove from heat and stir in 2 cups of shredded cheese. Mix in half of bacon and season to taste. Top with cheese, bacon and green onion.

Spinach Salad
9 ounces fresh baby spinach
5 ounces grape tomatoes, halved, about 16
2 ounces red onion, sliced thin
2 hard-boiled eggs, sliced
1/2 pound bacon, cooked until crisp and crumbled
1/2 cup ranch dressing
2 small avocados, mashed

In a small bowl, combined avocadoes and ranch dressing. In another bowl, combine all ingredients and top with dressing.

Tuna Melt
Tuna salad
12 ounces canned tuna, drained
4 eggs, hard boiled and coarsely chopped
1/4 cup sugar free sweet pickle relish
1/4 cup mayonnaise

1 tablespoon chives, minced
Salt and pepper, to taste
1 large tomato
2 ounces cheddar or American cheese, shredded

Mix all ingredients for tuna salad together and put in refrigerator overnight or for at least 6 hours.

Line a cooking sheet with foil and spray with cooking spray. Slice tomato and place on foil. Top with tuna salad mixture. Add shredded cheese. Place in oven on broil for several minutes or until cheese is melted.

Chicken Pesto Salad
2 Cups cooked chicken breast, chopped
1 medium stalk celery, finely chopped
1/3 Cup mayonnaise
1/3 Cup chopped white onion
2 Tablespoons chopped fresh parsley
2 Tablespoons jarred pesto
1/4 Teaspoon salt
1/8 Teaspoon ground black pepper

Combine all ingredients and serve with cherry tomatoes or plain.

Chicken Lettuce Wraps
8 oz skinless, boneless chicken thighs, ground
1/4 cup water chestnuts, chopped fine
1/4 cup dried shiitake mushrooms
1 tbsp soy sauce
1/4 tsp dark soy sauce
1/2 tsp oyster sauce
1 1/2 tsp sesame oil
1 tbsp rice wine or dry sherry
1/2 tsp sugar
freshly ground white pepper, to taste
2 cloves garlic, finely chopped
6 iceberg lettuce leaves, rinsed (careful not to break)

Soak mushrooms in hot water for a few minutes to soften. Remove stems and chop. Combine soy sauces, sesame oil, rice wine, sugar and pepper in a small bowl. Mix chicken, mushrooms and water chestnuts in a bowl. Pour sauce mixture over chicken and let sit for 15 minutes. Sauté garlic in a medium skillet for 3 minutes. Add in chicken mixture and cook until done. Scoop cooked chicken mixture onto each lettuce leaf. Roll and serve.

BLT Wraps
4 slices lean bacon (pork or turkey) cooked and chopped
1 medium tomato, diced
1 tbsp light mayonnaise
3 large iceberg lettuce leaves
fresh cracked pepper (optional)

Cook bacon, chop and set aside. Shred 1 piece of the lettuce. Place shredded lettuce on each of the remaining leaves. Add tomatoes and season with salt and pepper if desired. Add bacon pieces. Roll and serve.

No-Chip Nachos
½ pound ground beef, cooked and drained
½ cup shredded cheese
3 lettuce leaves
½ can mushroom pieces
½ cup shredded cabbage
¼ cup green jalapeno slices
¼ cup black olives, sliced
purple onion
2 cherry tomatoes cut in half

Place lettuce on a plate and top with hamburger. Add mushrooms, cabbage, jalapenos, olives and onion. Top with shredded cheese. Microwave for 30 seconds. Top with tomatoes.

Dinner

Beef Stroganoff
1 ¼ pounds skirt steak or beef tenderloin, cut into 2 x 1 strips
1/8 teaspoon salt
1/8 teaspoon pepper
2 tablespoons canola oil
1 tablespoon butter
½ cup finely chopped onion
3 ounce small white mushrooms
¼ cup dry red wine
1 cup beef broth (not low sodium)
¼ cup sour cream
1 teaspoon Dijon mustard

Sprinkle meat with salt and pepper. Heat oil in skillet over high heat. Brown beef strips. Place browned meat on an oven safe platter and put in oven at 185 degrees or warm setting. Add butter to skillet and sauté onions until clear. Add in mushrooms and cook for another 10 minutes or until liquid is gone. Add in the wine and cook for 5 minutes. Add in the beef broth and allow mixture to cool for another 10 minutes. Mushrooms should be coated with thick sauce. Mix sour cream and mustard into the skillet before adding meat strips. Cook for an additional 2 to 3 minutes on low heat.

Chicken Enchilada Zucchini Boats
olive oil spray
2 garlic cloves, minced
1 or 2 tbsp chipotle chile in adobo sauce, more if you like it spicy
1-1/2 cups tomato sauce
1/2 tsp chipotle chili powder
1/2 tsp ground cumin
2/3 cup fat-free low-sodium chicken broth
salt and fresh pepper to taste

For the zucchini boats:
4 (about 32 oz total) medium zucchini

1 tsp oil
1/2 cup green onions, chopped
3 cloves garlic, crushed
1/2 cup diced green bell pepper
1/4 cup chopped cilantro
8 oz cooked shredded chicken breast
1 tsp cumin
1/2 tsp dried oregano
1/2 tsp chipotle chili powder
3 tbsp water or fat free chicken broth
1 tbsp tomato paste
salt and pepper to taste

Topping:
Cheese
Fresh cilantro

To make sauce, spray the bottom of a saucepan with oil. Sauté garlic for 3 minutes. Mix in remaining ingredients and let simmer for 10 minutes. Remove from heat and set aside.

Cut zucchini in half lengthwise. Use a spoon to scoop out the center of each boat and place in a small bowl. Place halved zucchini into a pot of boiling water and cook about 1 minute or until softened. Set aside.

In a large skillet, heat oil and add onions, garlic and pepper. Cook for 3 minutes. Add in chopped zucchini and cilantro and cool for an additional 4 minutes. Add in remaining spices and tomato paste and let simmer for 3 minutes. Mix in chicken and let cook for 3 more minutes.

In a shallow baking dish, pour half of the enchilada sauce to cover bottom. Place halved zucchini with bowl side up in the dish. Scoop chicken mixture into each zucchini half. Add 2 tablespoons of enchilada sauce to each boat and top with shredded cheese and cilantro. Cover dish with foil. Bake in oven at 400 degrees for 35 minutes.

Philly Cheese Steak
1 steak
1/4 cup onion, sliced or chopped, 1 1/2 ounces
1/2 green pepper, sliced or chopped, about 3 ounces
1/4 of a 4 ounce can mushrooms, drained
Butter or oil
Salt and pepper
1/2 ounce provolone cheese or Monterey jack cheese, sliced

Season and grill steak as desired. In a skillet, sauté onion, peppers and mushrooms in butter or oil. Spread veggies over steak and top with cheese.

Ranch Crusted Chicken
1 bag LC Breading and Crusting Mix-Check your gluten-free aisle at grocery store
1 1/2 tsp garlic powder
1/4 cup heavy white cream
1/4 cup ranch dressing
6-8 pounds of chicken breasts, rinsed and patted dry with paper towels

Mix garlic powder with crust mix in a Ziploc bag, paper bag or bowl. Mix cream and ranch dressing in a bowl. Dip the chicken breasts in the cream mixture and toss in bag filled with crust mix. Bake for 35 minutes at 350 degrees.

Mexican Pie
2 lbs. ground meat, cooked & drained
1/2 cup chopped onions
1/4 cup chopped green pepper
2 teaspoons chili powder
8 oz. shredded cheddar cheese
8 oz. can tomato sauce
1/2 teaspoon garlic powder
1/2 cup + 1 Tablespoon sour cream
1 egg white, beaten stiff

In a large skillet, place meat, onions, pepper, garlic powder, tomato sauce and chili powder. Simmer for 8 minutes. Place meat mixture in an 8x8 baking dish. In a small bowl, mix sour cream, cheese and egg white. Pour mixture over the meat and bake at 375 for 30 minutes.

Tilapia Parmesan
2 tilapia fillets (5 oz to 6 oz each - if frozen, be sure to thaw fully before cooking)
2 teaspoons light mayonnaise
2 teaspoons non-fat plain yogurt
1/4 cup shredded parmesan cheese
2 to 4 sprigs of fresh dill
1 tsp garlic powder or garlic salt, divided
black pepper
non-stick cooking spray

In a small bowl, mix mayo, yogurt and parmesan cheese. Place a layer of foil on a cookie sheet and spray with cooking spray. Place fillets on cookie sheet. Spread the mayo mixture over the fillets. Sprinkle fillets with dill, garlic salt and pepper. Broil fillets for 6 to 7 minutes. When parmesan starts to brown, watch fish closely to avoid overcooking.

Fake Tater Casserole
16 oz bag frozen cauliflower
2 T light butter with canola oil
4 oz cream cheese, softened
1 lb turkey bacon, cooked until crispy and crumbled
8 oz shredded sharp cheddar cheese, divided
2 T chopped green onions
2 T Water

Place cauliflower and water in a microwaveable bowl and heat for 10 to 15 minutes or until cauliflower is very soft. Mash cauliflower and stir in butter and cream cheese. Add in all but ½ cup of the shredded cheese, bacon and onions. Mix well. Spread mixture in a baking dish and sprinkle remaining cheese over the top. Bake at 350 degrees for 20 minutes.

Snacks

Zucchini Bread
2 large eggs
2 Tablespoons canola oil
1 Teaspoon vanilla extract
4.5 Ounce shredded zucchini (1 cup)
1 Cup golden flaxseed meal
2 Tablespoons low-carb vanilla protein powder (1oz)
1/3 Cup granular sugar substitute
3/4 Teaspoon baking powder
1/4 Teaspoon salt
1 1/2 Teaspoons ground cinnamon
1/8 Teaspoon ground allspice
1/8 Teaspoon nutmeg

Mix eggs, oil and vanilla in a small bowl. Add in zucchini. In a large bowl, combine the remaining ingredients. Mix wet ingredients into the dry ingredients. Pour mixture into a greased muffin pan. Cook for 25 minutes at 350 degrees.

Mozzarella Sticks
1 cup crushed pork rinds
1 egg, lightly beaten
16 pieces of string cheese
peanut oil (enough to fill a skillet 1/2")

Heat oil on high heat, use enough oil to get at least ½ inch in bottom of skillet. Beat egg in a bowl. Dip string cheese in egg mixture. Roll cheese sticks in crushed pork rinds. Use your hands to press crushed rinds to cheese. Place in oil and cook for 2 minutes before turning and cooking for an additional 2 to 4 minutes.

Broiled Peaches
Two 15-ounce cans peach halves canned in extra-light syrup.
2 tablespoons light margarine
2 teaspoons brown sugar substitute
Cinnamon

Drain the peaches. Place peaches with cut side up in a broiling pan. Put a small pat of butter in the center of each peach. Sprinkle with cinnamon and sugar. Put in oven on broil for 10 minutes.

Chocolate Ice Cream
3 Cups heavy cream
2 large eggs
2 large egg yolks
3/4 Cup unsweetened cocoa powder
3/4 Cup granular sugar substitute (sucralose)
1/4 Teaspoon salt
2 Teaspoons vanilla extract
1/2 Teaspoon almond extract

Heat cream in a saucepan over medium heat. Bring cream to a slow boil, stirring constantly. Remove from heat. In a large mixing bowl, combine egg yolks, eggs, cocoa powder, salt and sugar substitute. Use an electric mixer on medium to blend mixture together for 2 minutes. Add a cup of the cream to the egg mixture and blend. Pour the egg mixture into the saucepan with the remaining cream. Heat on medium heat for 2 minutes, gently stirring to keep from scorching. Remove from heat and add vanilla and almond extract. Refrigerate mixture for 2 hours. You can pour the mix into an ice cream maker or simply stir and place in freezer overnight.

Conclusion

Thank you again for purchasing this book!

You now have all the tools you will need to begin your journey to better health with the Atkins Diet plan. I trust the knowledge you have gained will be extremely valuable and rewarding on your quest for better health.

If you enjoyed this book, please take the time to share your thoughts and post a review on Amazon. I would greatly appreciate it!

Thank you and good luck!

PS: You may also be interested in my other books. Get them on Amazon today!

The Sugar Detox Solution: A Proven Strategy for Weight Loss, Improving Your Health and Feeling Great by Defeating Your Sugar Cravings and Addiction

DASH Diet Essentials: A Beginner's Guide to the DASH Diet with a Proven Lifestyle Plan and Delicious Recipes so You can Lower Your Blood Pressure, Lose Weight, Feel Great and Live a Healthy Life

These are all great resources I created to help you on your way to better health. It's part of my Healthy Life Series.

References

http://www.atkinsfoundation.org/about

http://www.atkins.com/Science/Science-Behind-Atkins.aspx

http://www.atkins.com/AtkinsDotCom/media/Master/Publis hed-Atkins-Supporting-Research-060413.pdf

http://www.healthline.com/health/atkins-diet

http://www.webmd.com/diet/high-protein-low-carbohydrate-diets

http://www.everythingatkins.net/inductionphase.html

http://lowcarbdiets.about.com/od/atkinsdiet/p/atkins1.htm

http://www.weightwatchers.com/util/art/index_art.aspx?tab num=1&art_id=8311&sc=128

http://www.cdc.gov/healthyweight/assessing/bmi/adult_bmi /english_bmi_calculator/bmi_calculator.html

http://www.atkins.com/Recipes.aspx

http://authoritynutrition.com/101-healthy-low-carb-recipes/

http://www.skinnytaste.com/2012/08/chicken-enchilada-stuffed-zucchini-boats.html

http://www.buzzfeed.com/christinebyrne/satisfying-low-carb-dinners#19almnh

http://www.genaw.com/lowcarb/recipes.html

http://www.skinnytaste.com/2007/07/low-carb-recipes.html

http://yourlighterside.com/low-carb-gluten-free-snacks-sandwiches-recipes/

http://recipes.sparkpeople.com/browse-results.asp?category=low+carb

http://www.atkins.com/Science/Articles---Library/Carbohydrates/What-are-Net-Carbs--%281%29.aspx

www.ingramcontent.com/pod-product-compliance
Lightning Source LLC
Chambersburg PA
CBHW070241290526
45789CB00004B/1721